HOW TO MANAGE YOUR PCOS SYMPTOMS

Healthy Lifestyle Changes for Polycystic Ovary Syndrome Wellness

Victoria S. Miller

Contents

INTRODUCTION TO POLYCYSTIC OVARY SYNDROME

What is Polycystic Ovary Syndrome?

Polycystic ovary syndrome (PCOS) is a hormonal imbalance that happens when your ovaries, which are the organs responsible for producing and releasing eggs, generate excess hormones.

If you have PCOS, your ovaries produce abnormally high quantities of androgens. This causes an imbalance in your reproductive hormones. As a result, PCOS patients often have irregular menstrual cycles, missed periods, and uncertain ovulation.

Small follicle cysts (fluid-filled sacs containing immature eggs) may be detected on your ovaries on ultrasound owing to a lack of ovulation (anovulation). However, despite the name "polycystic," it is not necessary to have cysts on your ovaries to have PCOS. The ovarian cysts are neither hazardous nor painful.

PCOS is one of the most prevalent causes of infertility in women and persons assigned female at birth (AFAB). It may also raise your chance of developing other health problems.

Signs of Polycystic Ovary Syndrome

The following are the most prevalent signs and symptoms of PCOS:

1. Irregular periods
An abnormal menstrual cycle could include missing periods or not menstruating at all. There is also a chance of heavy bleeding during periods.

2. Unusual hair growth

Excess facial hair or excessive hair growth on your arms, chest, and abdomen (hirsutism) may occur. This affects up to 70% of PCOS patients.

3. Acne

Acne may be caused by PCOS, particularly on the back, chest, and face. This acne may persist throughout your adolescence and be tough to treat.

4. Obesity

Obesity affects 40% to 80% of patients with PCOS, and they struggle to maintain a healthy weight.

5. Darkening of the skin

Patches of dark skin may appear, particularly in the creases of your neck, armpits, groin (between your legs), and beneath your breasts. This is referred to as acanthosis nigricans.

6. Cysts

On ultrasound, many patients with PCOS have ovaries that seem bigger or with numerous follicles (egg sac cysts).

7. Skin tags

Skin tags are little flaps of excess skin. They are often seen in the armpits or on the neck.

8. Thinning hair

People suffering from PCOS may have hair loss or become bald.

9. Infertility

PCOS is the most prevalent cause of infertility in people AFAB. Failure to ovulate on a regular or frequent basis might result in infertility.

PCOS can develop without any symptoms. Many people don't realize they have the condition until they have trouble becoming pregnant or start gaining weight for no apparent reason. It's also possible to have mild PCOS, which means that the symptoms are not severe enough to be noticed.

Causes of PCOS

The exact cause of PCOS is unknown. There is evidence that genetics is involved. Several other factors, most particularly obesity, also have a role in the cause of PCOS:

1. Increased amounts of male hormones known as androgens

High amounts of androgen hinder your ovaries from producing eggs, resulting in irregular menstrual cycles. Irregular ovulation may also result in the formation of tiny, fluid-filled sacs on your ovaries. Acne and excessive hair growth are also caused by increased amounts of androgens in women and people with AFAB.

2. Insulin resistance

When your insulin levels rise, your ovaries produce and release male hormones (androgens). Greater levels of male hormones suppress ovulation and are a factor in other PCOS symptoms. Your body processes glucose (sugar) and uses it for energy with the help of insulin. When your body does not correctly process insulin, you develop insulin resistance, which results in too much glucose levels in your blood. Although not all people with insulin resistance have high blood sugar or diabetes, insulin resistance may lead to diabetes. Obesity and being overweight may also lead to insulin resistance. Even if your blood glucose is normal, a high insulin level might suggest insulin resistance.

3. Low-grade inflammation

PCOS patients often experience persistent low-grade inflammation. Blood tests may be performed by your healthcare provider to detect levels of C-reactive protein (CRP) and white blood cells, which can indicate the degree of inflammation in your body.

DIAGNOSIS AND EFFECTS ON HEALTH

How PCOS is Diagnosed

PCOS is commonly diagnosed in women who have at least two of the following three symptoms:

- High amounts of androgen
- Irregular menstrual cycles
- Ovaries with cysts

Your doctor may ask you about your medical history as well as do a physical exam and several tests to help diagnose PCOS and rule out other causes of your symptoms.

1. Physical examination

Your blood pressure, body mass index (BMI), and waist size will be measured by your doctor. They will also examine your skin for excess hair on your face, chest, or back, as well as acne or skin discoloration.

2. Pelvic examination

Your doctor may do a pelvic exam to look for signs of excess male hormones (such as an enlarged clitoris) and to see whether your ovaries are big or swollen.

3. Pelvic ultrasound (sonogram)

This test uses sound waves to examine your ovaries for cysts and check the endometrium (uterine or womb lining).

4. Blood tests

Blood tests measure your androgen hormone levels, sometimes known as "male hormones." Your doctor will also look for other hormones associated with other common health issues that might be confused with PCOS, such as thyroid disease. Additionally, your doctor could examine your blood sugar and cholesterol levels.

How Does PCOS Affect Your Body?

1. Infertility

You must ovulate to become pregnant. Women who do not ovulate regularly do not release as many eggs to be fertilized. PCOS is one of the primary reasons for infertility in women.

2. Metabolic syndrome

Most women with PCOS are overweight or obese. Obesity and PCOS both increase your chances of:

- High blood sugar levels
- High blood pressure
- Low HDL "good" cholesterol
- High LDL "bad" cholesterol

Together, these factors are referred to as metabolic syndrome, and they raise the risk of:

- Cardiovascular disease
- Diabetes
- Stroke

3. Sleep apnea

This disorder causes repeated pauses in breathing throughout the night, disrupting sleep.

Sleep apnea is more frequent in overweight women, particularly if they also have PCOS. Women with both obesity and PCOS have 5 to 10 times increased risk of sleep apnea than those without PCOS.

4. Endometrial cancer

The uterine lining sheds during ovulation. The lining might accumulate if you do not ovulate every month.

Endometrial cancer risk can be increased by a thickened uterine lining.

5. Depression

Both hormonal changes and symptoms such as undesired hair growth may have a detrimental impact on your emotions. Many people with PCOS ultimately develop depression and anxiety.

PCOS AND RELATIONSHIPS

PCOS is a frustrating condition that can affect fertility, health, and emotional well-being in women. It is not unexpected that PCOS may have an impact on your relationship with your spouse, family, and friends.

Here are some of the factors that may have an impact on your relationships if you have PCOS, as well as what you can do about it.

1. Low self-esteem
PCOS may produce several distressing dermatological symptoms, including acne, hirsutism, abnormal hair growth or hair loss, and skin tags, in addition to producing reproductive problems such as irregular periods and trouble conceiving. It is also

linked to weight gain and endocrine issues such as diabetes. These bodily changes might impair your self-esteem and make you feel uneasy in your skin. You may also experience mood disorders such as anxiety and depression, which can have a negative impact on your self-esteem.

Remember that your family and friends adore you for who you are, not because your skin is flawless or your hair is flawless. After all, you don't care for your closest buddy for that reason, do you? Respect yourself and have faith that your loved ones love you just as much as you love them. If this becomes a persistent issue, consider consulting with a mental health expert to work through any negative ideas you may be having.

2. Weight changes
Many women with PCOS struggle to lose weight. If you've been struggling to lose any PCOS-related weight, you may feel resentful of friends who are slimmer or don't have to watch their weight. Many women described feeling constantly compared to their skinnier friends or being ashamed about their excess weight.

If your weight is a concern, get advice on lifestyle adjustments from a qualified dietitian who has expertise in treating women with PCOS.

3. Infertility and intimacy

Infertility, or difficulty getting pregnant, can have a significant impact on a couple's relationship. Being open about your private sexual life to medical experts might also have a negative impact on your intimacy. Even being told when to have sex and when to abstain takes away the spontaneity and fun of being in a relationship. Couples frequently fight during this period, especially given the financial and emotional strain of fertility treatment. If you believe your infertility is your fault, know that infertility is common and it is not something to be ashamed of.

Infertility does not have to be the end of your relationship with your partner. You can do a lot to restore or maintain the intimacy and spontaneity of your sexual relationship. Work with your partner to come up with fun ways to initiate sex and make time to appreciate each other outside of the bedroom, it doesn't have to be inside the bedroom. Making time for each other can help improve your relationship and make trying to conceive more fulfilling.

If you believe that having PCOS is negatively impacting your relationships with others, it may be time to consult with an individual psychotherapist or a couples' counselor for assistance.

PCOS AND PREGNANCY

Becoming pregnant can be more challenging if you have been diagnosed with PCOS. Should you conceive, you may face a higher risk of complications during pregnancy, as well as throughout labor and delivery.

Individuals with PCOS are thrice as likely to experience a miscarriage in comparison to those without the condition. They are also at an increased risk for conditions such as preeclampsia, gestational diabetes, delivering a larger infant, and preterm birth, which could complicate delivery, potentially necessitating a cesarean section.

Risks for Expectant Mothers with PCOS

Conceiving can be a difficult journey for those with PCOS due to hormonal imbalances. Obesity is more common among women with PCOS, and many require assisted reproductive technologies to conceive. Research indicates that about 60 percent of women with PCOS are obese, and nearly 14 percent need fertility assistance.

PCOS elevates the risk of several health issues throughout a woman's life, including insulin resistance, type 2 diabetes, elevated cholesterol, hypertension, cardiovascular disease, stroke, sleep apnea, and possibly a heightened risk of endometrial cancer.

For expectant mothers, PCOS introduces additional risks such as preeclampsia, a serious condition endangering both mother and baby. The preferred intervention for preeclampsia symptoms is the delivery of the baby and placenta. Doctors will weigh the risks and benefits regarding the timing of delivery, based on symptom severity and the baby's gestational age. Close monitoring is essential if preeclampsia develops. Other concerns include pregnancy-induced hypertension and gestational diabetes.

Gestational diabetes may result in a larger baby, complicating delivery, such as increasing the risk of shoulder dystocia during labor. Most PCOS symptoms during pregnancy can be managed with vigilant monitoring and, if necessary, insulin to maintain stable blood sugar levels.

Risks for the Infant

PCOS complicates pregnancy, necessitating increased monitoring for both mother and child.

Potential risks for the baby associated with PCOS include:

- Preterm birth
- Being large for gestational age
- Miscarriage
- Lower Apgar scores

Women with PCOS often deliver by cesarean due to the tendency to have larger infants, and other labor and delivery complications may arise.

Conceiving with PCOS

Many women may not discover they have PCOS until attempting to conceive, as the condition can go undetected. If you have been trying to conceive naturally for more than a year without success, consider consulting your physician for testing.

Your doctor can assist in formulating a plan to enhance your chances of conception. Strategies such as weight loss, a nutritious diet, and possibly medication can improve fertility prospects.

Strategies for Conceiving with PCOS

PCOS does not preclude pregnancy; it may simply require additional assistance. There are numerous actions you can take, both at home and with medical intervention, to manage PCOS symptoms and increase the likelihood of a healthy pregnancy.

Conceiving with PCOS involves steps similar to those recommended for women without PCOS aiming for a healthy pregnancy.

1. Consult your doctor to assess your weight and body mass index (BMI). A healthy body weight and composition are crucial. If you are overweight, discuss with your physician the amount of weight loss needed before conception.

2. Implement a nutritious diet and exercise regimen. Opt for healthier food selections and increase physical activity.

3. Utilize ovulation calendars or apps to track menstrual cycles. This will help identify your most fertile days.

4. Regularly monitor blood sugar levels. Balanced blood sugar is vital for conception, a healthy pregnancy, and the future health of your child.

Maintaining a Healthy Weight

While there is an association between being overweight and PCOS, not all women with the condition are overweight. Nevertheless, losing even 5% of your body weight can enhance fertility and reduce other PCOS symptoms if you are carrying extra weight.

Incorporate daily exercise, such as walking or using a standing desk instead of sitting, and build muscle through light weightlifting to mitigate PCOS symptoms and improve overall health.

Eating for Health

Proper nutrition is essential for anyone trying to conceive. Replace sugary snacks, simple carbohydrates, and unhealthy fats with healthier alternatives, including:

- Fresh and cooked fruits and vegetables
- Whole grains such as brown rice, oats, and barley
- Legumes like beans and lentils

- Poultry and fish

Certain vitamins and minerals are crucial for a healthy pregnancy and fetal development. Discuss with your doctor the most suitable supplements for your needs. Supplements that may aid fertility include folic acid (vitamin B9), vitamins B6, B12, C, D, E, and coenzyme Q10.

Balancing Blood Sugar Levels

PCOS can lead to elevated blood sugar levels or type 2 diabetes, potentially affecting fertility.

PCOS may alter insulin utilization in the body, the hormone responsible for moving glucose from the bloodstream into cells for energy. PCOS can reduce insulin sensitivity, making its job more challenging.

Stabilizing blood sugar levels can assist in conception. A diet rich in fiber, protein, and healthy fats, along with regular exercise and strength training, can improve insulin sensitivity.

In some cases, medications like metformin, a common diabetes drug, may be prescribed to enhance insulin efficiency and aid in conception with PCOS.

Monitoring blood sugar levels at home and undergoing tests such as random blood sugar tests, overnight fasting tests, oral glucose tolerance tests, and hemoglobin A1C tests are important if you have high blood sugar levels or diabetes.

Medications

With PCOS, the body may produce an excess of both testosterone and estrogen. Imbalanced hormones can complicate conception. Your doctor may suggest prescription medications to help regulate your hormone levels.

Medications that may aid in conceiving with PCOS include:

- Metformin for insulin level regulation
- Clomiphene citrate (Clomid) to balance estrogen levels

- Birth control pills to regulate estrogen and testosterone levels (before fertility treatments)
- Fertility medications to stimulate the ovaries to release more eggs

Fertility Assistance

In vitro fertilization (IVF) may be necessary to assist with conception in PCOS cases. Your fertility specialist will conduct a thorough evaluation, which may include additional blood tests, ultrasound scans, and a physical examination.

IVF is a process that can span months or years, regardless of PCOS status. However, studies suggest that women with PCOS have a high success rate of conceiving through IVF.

Some clinical studies have shown that women with PCOS who took birth control pills before IVF had improved outcomes. Additional medications may be needed to balance hormones and prepare the body for IVF.

For all women, the initial step in IVF is to maintain a balanced diet and engage in regular exercise to achieve a healthy weight. Women with PCOS at a healthy weight have twice the chance of conceiving through IVF compared to those who are obese.

Before considering IVF, your doctor may suggest a less expensive alternative known as intrauterine insemination (IUI). This method enhances the likelihood of pregnancy by directly introducing a concentrated amount of sperm closer to the egg.

TREATMENTS

PCOS cannot be cured, but treatments can help you manage the symptoms and reduce your risk of long-term health problems.

Medical Treatments

1. Combination birth control pills
Pills that contain both estrogen and progestin reduce androgen production and regulate estrogen. Hormone control may reduce your risk of endometrial cancer as well as correct irregular bleeding, excess hair growth, and acne.

2. Progestin therapy
Taking progestin for 10 to 14 days every 1 to 2 months can control your periods and protect against

endometrial cancer. This progestin therapy does not enhance androgen levels and won't prevent pregnancy.

Your healthcare provider may advise you to do the following to help you ovulate and get pregnant:

3. Clomiphene

Clomiphene, an oral anti-estrogen medication, is taken during the first part of your menstrual cycle.

4. Metformin

Metformin, an oral type 2 diabetes medication, improves insulin resistance and reduces insulin levels. If you do not get pregnant while taking clomiphene, your doctor may advise you to take metformin to help you ovulate. If you have prediabetes, metformin may help you lose weight and reduce the progression to type 2 diabetes.

5. Gonadotropins

These hormone medicines are administered through injection.

If necessary, see your doctor about treatments that may assist you in becoming pregnant. In vitro fertilization, for example, may be a possibility.

Your doctor may advise you to do the following to lower excessive hair growth or improve acne:

6. Birth control pills

These pills reduce testosterone production, which can cause excessive hair growth and acne.

7. Spironolactone (Aldactone)

This medicine blocks androgen's effects on the skin, including excessive hair growth and acne. Because spironolactone can cause birth abnormalities, it is essential to use effective birth control while taking this medicine. This medication is not advised if you are pregnant or want to become pregnant.

8. Eflornithine (Vaniqa)

This cream may help to reduce the growth of facial hair.

9. Hair removal

Hair removal methods include electrolysis and laser hair removal. Electrolysis is carried out by inserting a small needle into each hair follicle. The needle emits an electric current pulse. The current damages, then destroys the follicle. Laser hair removal is a medical procedure that uses a focused beam of light to remove unwanted hair. You may need numerous electrolysis or laser hair removal treatment. Other options include shaving, plucking, or using creams that destroy unwanted hair. However, they are just temporary, and hair may thicken as it grows back.

10. Acne treatment
Medications, such as pills and topical creams or gels, may help improve acne. Consult your doctor about your choices.

Natural Treatments

1. Dietary modifications
Eating the right meals and avoiding specific ingredients may help to manage your symptoms. A healthy diet may help you control your hormones and menstrual cycle. Consuming highly processed, preserved foods may lead to inflammation and insulin resistance.

It all comes down to whole foods

Artificial sugars, hormones, and preservatives are not found in whole foods. These foods are as close to their natural, unprocessed state as possible. Whole foods that you may include in your diet include fruits, vegetables, whole grains, and legumes.

Your endocrine system can regulate your blood sugar levels more effectively without hormones and preservatives.

Balance your carbohydrate and protein consumption

Protein and carbohydrates both affect your energy and hormone levels. Eating protein promotes your body's production of insulin. Unprocessed, high-carbohydrate foods may boost insulin sensitivity. Rather than attempting a low-carb diet, concentrate on eating enough healthy protein.
The best plant-based protein sources are nuts, legumes, and whole grains.

Aim for anti-inflammatory

According to research, PCOS is characterized by low-level chronic inflammation. Anti-inflammatory foods may assist to ease your symptoms.

Consider the Mediterranean diet as a choice. Anti-inflammatory foods include olive oil, tomatoes, leafy greens, fatty fish like mackerel and tuna, and tree nuts.

Increase your iron intake

During menstruation, some women with PCOS experience heavy bleeding. This may lead to anemia or iron deficiency. If your doctor has diagnosed you with either condition, discuss with them how you might increase your iron intake. They may advise you to include iron-rich foods like spinach, eggs, and broccoli in your diet.

You should not increase your iron intake without first speaking with your doctor. Too much iron intake might raise your risk of complications.

Increase your magnesium intake

Magnesium-rich PCOS foods include spinach, bananas, almonds, and cashews.

Include some fiber to aid digestion

A fiber-rich diet may help improve digestion. Fiber-rich foods include lentils, broccoli, Brussels sprouts, pears, and avocados.

Refrain from coffee

Caffeine intake might be associated with changes in estrogen levels and hormone behavior. Try a decaf option, like herbal tea, to boost your energy. The probiotic properties of kombucha may also be of benefit.

If you can't go without a caffeine boost, try green tea instead. Insulin resistance is improved by drinking green tea. It may also aid in weight control in women with PCOS.

2. Supplements

Supplements claim to aid with PCOS-related hormone regulation, insulin resistance, and inflammation.

Before using any supplement, consult your doctor. Some of them might interfere with other PCOS treatments and medications.

Inositol

Inositol is a B vitamin that may help improve insulin resistance. It has also been shown to aid fertility in certain instances of PCOS.

Chromium

Chromium supplements may help with PCOS by improving your body mass index.
They may also help your body metabolize sugar, which may help steady insulin resistance.

Cinnamon

Cinnamon is derived from the bark of cinnamon trees. Cinnamon extract has been proven to have a positive effect on insulin resistance. Cinnamon may also help people with PCOS regulate their menstrual cycles.

Turmeric

Curcumin is the active ingredient in turmeric. Turmeric has the potential to reduce insulin resistance and act as an anti-inflammatory agent.

Zinc

Zinc is a trace element that might improve your fertility and immune system. Zinc supplements may help with excessive or undesired hair growth and alopecia.

To obtain more zinc in your diet, consume red meat, beans, tree nuts, and shellfish.

Evening primrose oil

Evening primrose oil has been used to treat period discomfort and irregular menstruation. It may also help improve cholesterol levels and oxidative stress, both of which are associated with PCOS.

Combined vitamin D and calcium

Vitamin D is an essential hormone for your endocrine system. Vitamin D deficiency is common in women with PCOS. Vitamin D and calcium may help with irregular periods and ovulation.

Cod liver oil

Cod liver oil is rich in omega-3 fatty acids and contains vitamins D and A. These acids may help improve menstruation regularity and help you lose fat around your waist.

Berberine

Berberine is a Chinese medicine to help with insulin resistance. Berberine may boost your metabolism and balance your body's endocrine reactions if you have PCOS.

3. Adaptogen herbs

When your body is unable to control insulin, it might produce an increase in male sex hormones known as androgens. Adaptogen herbs are said to help your body in balancing these hormones. Some adaptogen herbs also claim to alleviate other PCOS symptoms, such as irregular periods.

Before using any herbal supplement, exercise care and consult your doctor, since the FDA has not verified their claims.

Maca root

The maca plant's root is a traditional herb used to increase fertility and libido. Maca root may aid in hormone balance and cortisol reduction. It may also aid in the treatment of depression, which is a symptom of PCOS.

Ashwagandha

Ashwagandha is sometimes referred to as "Indian ginseng." It may help regulate cortisol levels, which may improve stress and PCOS symptoms.

Holy basil

Holy basil, also known as tulsi, addresses chemical and metabolic stress. It is known as the "queen of herbs." Holy basil may help decrease blood sugar, prevent weight gain, and lessen cortisol levels.

Licorice root

Glycyrrhizin, a compound found in the root of the licorice plant, has various unique qualities. Anti-inflammatory properties of licorice root have been proposed. It aids in the metabolism of sugar and the control of hormones.

4. Probiotics

Probiotics are useful for more than simply digestion and gut health. They may be beneficial in the treatment of PCOS. They also can decrease inflammation and control sex hormones such as androgen and estrogen.

Take probiotic supplements and consume probiotic foods such as kimchi and kombucha.

5. Keep a healthy weight
Keeping a healthy weight may help minimize insulin resistance, regulate your period, and lower your risk of PCOS-associated disorders.

If you are overweight, some research suggests that losing weight gradually using a low-calorie diet is a good first-line treatment for PCOS.

6. Maintain a healthy exercise routine
Maintaining a healthy weight requires exercise. However, too much exercise might disrupt your hormones, so see your doctor to find a healthy balance.

Gentle, low-impact workouts such as yoga or Pilates may be done for extended periods. Swimming and gentle aerobic exercise are also recommended. High-intensity interval training and long-distance running may also help improve PCOS symptoms.

Consult your doctor about the type of exercise that would be most beneficial to you.

7. Maintain proper sleep hygiene

Sleep lowers stress and helps to regulate cortisol, which helps to balance your hormones. However, sleep disruptions are twice as prevalent in women with PCOS. Improve your sleep hygiene by doing the following:

- Attempt to get 8 to 10 hours of sleep every night
- Establish a consistent nighttime routine
- Before going to bed, avoid stimulants and rich, fatty meals

8. Reduce stress

Cortisol levels may be regulated by reducing stress. Many of the strategies mentioned above, such as yoga, getting adequate sleep, and avoiding caffeine, may help to reduce stress.

Taking walks outdoors and making time in your life for relaxation and self-care might also help you feel less stressed.

9. Avoid or limit the use of endocrine disruptors
Chemicals or ingredient compounds that interfere with or obstruct your body's normal hormonal reactions are known as endocrine disruptors.

Some endocrine disruptors mimic female and male sex hormones, leading to confusion in your reproductive system. This might raise your chances of developing PCOS symptoms.

They're often found in canned foods, soaps, and cosmetics. Endocrine disruptors that are commonly used include:

- Dioxins
- Phthalates
- Pesticides
- BPA
- Glycol ethers

10. Think about acupuncture
There is adequate research to support acupuncture as an alternative treatment for PCOS. Acupuncture may aid in the treatment of PCOS by:

- Boosting blood flow to your ovaries

- Lowering cortisol levels
- Helping with weight loss
- Improving your insulin sensitivity

If you're contemplating any of the natural PCOS treatment options listed above, consult with your doctor to develop a treatment plan.

While herbal supplements and other treatments may aid in PCOS treatment, they are not a replacement for a tailored, ongoing dialogue with your doctor about your symptoms.

PCOS AND MENOPAUSE

Menopause is caused by a steady decrease in female hormone levels. PCOS symptoms may continue into menopause. Polycystic ovary syndrome and menopause are both related to hormones, however, menopause does not cure PCOS. When you enter menopause, you may still have certain PCOS symptoms in addition to menopause symptoms.

How Does PCOS and Menopause Influence Hormones?

Women who have PCOS tend to have greater amounts of male hormones, including testosterone. PCOS also causes your body to be less responsive to insulin.

This results in high blood sugar levels. High blood sugar levels might increase male hormones, even more, exacerbating your PCOS symptoms.

Women with PCOS may have low amounts of the female hormone progesterone. Progesterone aids in the regulation of menstruation and the maintenance of a pregnancy.

Years before menopause, your body starts to generate less estrogen and progesterone. Ovulation ultimately stops due to a reduction in female hormones. When you haven't had a menstrual cycle in a year, you've entered menopause.

PCOS and menopause both alter progesterone levels in your blood, but they affect your hormones in different ways. As a result, menopause does not treat or cure PCOS.

Perimenopause Symptoms

When you approach perimenopause and menopause, you can still have PCOS symptoms. Perimenopause is the time before menopause when symptoms such as hot flashes and irregular cycles are common. Your hormone levels begin to alter in preparation for menopause during perimenopause. Perimenopause may last several years. When you haven't had a period for 12 months, you're considered to be in menopause.

Perimenopause usually begins in your forties or fifties. Menopause occurs at an average age of 51. Women with PCOS often enter menopause two years later than those without PCOS.

Because PCOS does not go away with menopause, you may continue to have symptoms. Some PCOS symptoms are similar to perimenopause symptoms. That may make it challenging for women to be newly diagnosed with PCOS during perimenopause

Perimenopause Symptoms

- Alterations in sex drive
- Irregular periods or missed periods
- Night sweating and hot flashes
- Infertility
- Pain and discomfort during intercourse

- Mood swings
- Sleeping problems
- Thinning hair on the head, particularly in middle age
- Undesired hair growth
- Urinary incontinence

- Infections of the vaginal and urinary tract
- Vaginal dryness and vaginal tissue thinning
- Weight gain

Managing PCOS in Perimenopause

Techniques for managing PCOS symptoms might also help with certain perimenopause symptoms.

1. Maintain a healthy weight

2. Improve your sleeping habits

3. Relieve hot flashes

4. Medications

PCOS AND EXERCISE

How Essential is Exercise for PCOS?

Regular exercise is essential for everyone, but it is particularly important for individuals with PCOS. Due to insulin resistance, those with PCOS are at a greater risk of obesity and diabetes, and losing weight may be difficult. There is a link between a lack of physical exercise and excessive body weight, and both may contribute to insulin resistance. Exercise, along with a balanced diet, can help you lose weight. Another advantage of exercising is that it helps to balance your hormones and reduce your testosterone levels. This will ease PCOS symptoms like excessive hair growth and acne. The following are some of the benefits of exercise for PCOS patients:

1. Balancing your hormones

Exercising helps to lower estrogen and insulin and increase endorphins.

2. Boosting your mood

As a result of hormone imbalances and PCOS symptoms, PCOS patients may be more prone to depression. Endorphins (happy hormones) are released as a result of regular exercise.

3. Improving autonomic function and inflammatory pattern

Exercise has been demonstrated in studies to enhance autonomic function (which controls involuntary body functions) as well as inflammatory patterns (the majority of persons with PCOS have increased levels of chronic inflammation).

4. Helping with weight loss

When you have PCOS, it might be difficult to lose weight. Losing weight will be easier if you combine daily exercise with a healthy eating plan.

5. Improving your sleep quality

Exercise may help you sleep soundly. PCOS patients are more likely to suffer from sleep apnea, snoring, and other sleep disorders. Obesity exacerbates these issues further.

6. Lowering your diabetes risk
Cardio exercise may increase your insulin response.

7. Aiding with cholesterol management
Women with PCOS are more likely to have elevated cholesterol, which may be reduced by exercising and a healthy diet.

8. Reduced risk of cardiovascular disease
You are also more prone to hypertension and cardiovascular diseases. Exercise will enhance your heart health.

What is the Best PCOS Exercise?

1. Consistent cardiovascular exercises
A consistent cardiovascular exercise is one in which the intensity of the exercise remains constant throughout the session. Walking, running, swimming, cycling, and hiking are examples of such activities. Even 30 minutes every day will help.

Cardiovascular exercise is beneficial for women with PCOS since they are at a greater risk of insulin resistance and weight gain. Cardiovascular exercise improves insulin sensitivity and prevents the effects of cholesterol deposition in the arteries, which may contribute to high blood pressure, heart disease, and type 2 diabetes. This form of exercise will also improve your mood and help you lose weight.

2. High-intensity interval training

HIIT (high-intensity interval training) is a mix of brief bursts of very-high-intensity cardio exercise followed by the same period or longer amount of rest. For example, one minute of running followed by one or two minutes of jogging or walking. Doing this for 10 minutes is a HIIT exercise.

Short aerobic bursts in HIIT are excellent for people with PCOS. The key benefit of HIIT is that it allows you to improve your cardiovascular fitness quicker by working harder rather than longer.

3. Strength training

Strength training uses your own body weight, resistance bands, or weights to build muscle. Resistance training was shown to be more successful than other forms of exercise in lowering the Free

Androgen Index (testosterone levels) in women with PCOS in a trial evaluating several types of exercise for PCOS. Strength training at both 'vigorous' and moderate intensities had beneficial outcomes, and the more often you performed it, the better.

Push-ups and tricep dips, for example, increase muscle and upper body strength while improving insulin function and burning calories long after you've done the exercise.

4. Mind-body exercises

As a result of their symptoms, women with PCOS often feel depressed, stressed, and anxious, and one research discovered that women with PCOS who were overweight had a greater degree of depression. Other PCOS symptoms might be exacerbated by stress. Mind-body activities such as yoga, tai chi, and pilates may assist to relieve stress while also burning calories, which can help with weight loss (when combined with a healthy diet and regular cardio exercise).

7 Days PCOS Exercise Plan

Here's a sample workout plan to help you get started with PCOS exercise. This plan is intended for those who are just starting with physical activity.

If you are already active, be sure that you are not overexerting yourself.

Always strive to include a different type of exercise in your weekly regimen. It will assist you in doing exercises on various sections of your body.

This helps to grow and strengthen various muscle groups while also providing general balance.

DAY 1: Brisk walk for 30 minutes. Continue to breathe deeply through your nose. At all times, avoid breathing through your mouth.

DAY 2: Yoga for 15 minutes - include various yoga postures such as butterfly stance, moving the grinding wheel, and cobra pose.

- 4-5 cycles of Sun Salutation

- 10 mins of Deep Breathing exercises

DAY 3: Brisk walk for 30 minutes. Continue to breathe deeply through your nose. At all times, avoid breathing through your mouth.

DAY 4: 30-40 minutes of brisk walking, swimming, or bicycling.

Alternatively, you may conduct a 10-minute cycling motion in bed while keeping your legs raised. Also, include 10 minutes of breathing exercises.

DAY 5: Yoga for 15 minutes - include various yoga postures such as butterfly stance, moving the grinding wheel, and cobra pose.

- 4-5 cycles of Sun Salutation
- 10 mins of Deep Breathing exercises

DAY 6: 10-20 cycles of squat

- 5-10 minutes of jumping jacks or rope skipping
- 20 cycles of lunge

DAY 7: Brisk walk for 30 minutes. Continue to breathe deeply through your nose. At all times, avoid breathing through your mouth.

How to Stick to a Workout Routine

It would be wonderful if you could work out today.

It would be even better if you worked out again the following day.

It would be ideal if you began and maintained a workout plan. (This is our aim!)

If we could, we would all work out most days of the week. But that is difficult. Time, schedules, motivation, and how you're feeling... are all factors that might get in your way.

So, how do we devise a plan and stick to it? Forming an exercise habit is not always easy, and it takes time and consistency before it becomes usual.

1. Link your habits

According to some studies, a great way to form a new habit is to link it to an existing one. Consider this: "Every time I ________, I will __________."

Consider combining something you do every day with a workout. When you clean your teeth, you could perform a wall sit or squats. Perform 20 jumping jacks and hold a plank for 20–30 seconds (the last five seconds should make you feel like quitting) while you wait for the shower to warm up.

Consider that you want to 'earn' your shower! Nothing like a nice, refreshing shower after a good sweat.

2. Balance before bed

Incorporate a balancing posture or a yoga pose into your sleep routine to create a more physically active lifestyle. Take a minute before going to bed to practice balance and calm.

These postures combine a mind-body connection, promote concentration, and may assist you in unwinding at the end of the day.

3. Imagine the action

Imagine yourself doing the workouts. Consider yourself to be someone who loves exercise and movement. Use all of your senses to make this even more powerful.

What will you see, smell, or hear during an enjoyable physical workout? Think of how you will feel afterward: sweaty, accomplished, and powerful.

4. Find your groove

Music may be a tremendous motivator as well. Create an entertaining playlist! Add music you like and only listen to them when working out, so they seem like a reward. Music may stimulate your senses and put you in the mood to exercise.

5. Watch TV while working out

Maybe you're seeking a distraction? If you're having a particularly demotivating day, you may perform these exercises while watching your favorite program on TV.

Just be careful not to get too distracted that you lose the correct form!

The Best PCOS Exercise Suggestion

In the end, this is what matters:

Pay attention to your body and do what feels right

Kick it if it's a kickboxing class! Do some yoga if you need a restorative day. It doesn't matter if it's hopping on your exercise bike, strength training, or a spinning class...whatever you can keep up in your hectic schedule and love doing is exactly what's good for you.

Congratulations if you're just starting with exercising! Even if you're unclear what to do, simply get started. The desire to move is an excellent starting point. Experiment, have fun, and discover what you like and what new physical activities you can add (and enjoy) to your life.

An extra benefit? You'll probably notice that your mental health improves alongside your physical health!

Exercising when you have PCOS has been demonstrated to improve a wide range of physical (and mental) symptoms! Realize that your efforts will be rewarded in the end.

The sooner you take charge of your physical health and fitness, the sooner you will be able to manage your symptoms rather than feeling as if PCOS has power over you.

PCOS-FRIENDLY RECIPES

1. Pumpkin Pancakes

Total time: 35 minutes
Servings: 2

Ingredients

- 4 eggs
- 1/2 cup pumpkin puree
- 1 teaspoon vanilla extract
- 1 teaspoon Ground Ceylon cinnamon
- 1 teaspoon pumpkin pie spice
- 1/2 teaspoon baking soda
- 1/8 teaspoon salt
- 2 tablespoons coconut flour (non-compulsory, incase your batter is too runny)
- 1 tablespoon Ghee (for the batter)

- 2 tablespoons Ghee (for frying pancakes)
- 1/2 cup coconut yogurt
- 1 cup frozen berries

Instructions

Step 1

In a large bowl, combine the eggs, pumpkin puree, vanilla extract, cinnamon, pie spice, baking soda, and salt. Whisk and mix until the mixture is entirely smooth.

Step 2

The thickness or runniness of the batter will be determined by the pumpkin puree and eggs used, so some trial and error may be necessary to get the desired consistency. In general, a little runnier combination than you are used to is preferable. If the batter needs to be thickened, add 1-2 tablespoons of coconut flour and let it sit for 10 minutes.

Step 3

Preheat a large skillet on medium-low. To complete the batter, quickly melt the ghee and stir it into the mixture before returning the skillet to the heat.

Step 4

Add a good quantity of ghee to the skillet and pour your batter in to make pancakes.

Step 5

When a few bubbles form, turn the pancakes over and cook until the second side is cooked through. Repeat until all of the batter is finished.

Step 6

If your pancakes are burnt on the outside and undercooked on the inside, reduce the heat and cook them slower. It may take some practice to get them correctly.

Step 7

Top the pancakes with yogurt and berries.

2. Swiss Chard Quiche

Total time: 50 minutes
Servings: 6

Ingredients

- 2 tablespoons olive oil
- 12 oz bacon or pork belly, diced
- 1 onion, diced
- 3 cups Swiss chard, stems detached, roughly chopped
- 1 zucchini, diced
- 10 eggs
- 1/3 cup canned coconut milk
- 3/4 teaspoon salt
- 1/4 teaspoon black pepper

Instructions

Step 1

Preheat the oven to 350°F (180°C) and lightly oil a 10" (25 cm) pie dish.

Step2

Add a little olive oil to a large skillet using medium heat and fry the bacon and onions for 8-10 minutes before transferring to the pie dish. Leave as much fat in the skillet as possible to let the vegetable cook.

Step 3

While the skillet is still hot, add the Swiss chard and zucchini and cook until tender. Transfer to the pie dish, leaving any excess water in the skillet.

Step 4

In a large bowl, whisk the eggs, coconut milk, salt, and pepper. Pour into the dish and cover the bacon/vegetable mixture.

Step 5

Bake in the oven for 30 minutes, or until the egg is completely set.

Step 6

Allow for a 15-minute cooling period before serving with hot sauce, sugar-free ketchup, or nutritional yeast.

Step 7

Keep any leftovers in a tightly sealed container in the refrigerator for up to 4 days.

---

3. Shrimp Fried Rice

Total time: 20 minutes
Servings: 4

Ingredients

- 2 tablespoons coconut oil
- 20 oz fresh shrimp, peeled, deveined
- 2 teaspoons garlic, minced
- 1 onion, finely diced
- 1 zucchini, finely diced
- 2 cups mushroom, finely diced
- 2 carrots, finely diced
- 6 cups cauliflower, riced
- 3 tablespoons coconut aminos
- 3 tablespoons Gluten-free tamari sauce
- 1 tablespoon fish sauce
- 1/4 teaspoon salt
- 1/4 teaspoon black pepper

- 4 scallions, chopped

Instructions

Step 1

In a large skillet using medium heat, heat the coconut oil. Add the shrimp and cook for 5 minutes.

Step 2

Set the shrimp aside, then add garlic, onion, zucchini, mushrooms, and carrots and cook for 5 minutes, stirring periodically.

Step3

Put the vegetables aside, then add the riced cauliflower to the skillet and cook for 5 minutes. If necessary, add a bit of extra coconut oil.

Step 4

When the riced cauliflower is done, put back the cooked vegetables and shrimp to the skillet.

Step 5

Add the coconut aminos, tamari sauce, and fish sauce and cook for 2 minutes, stirring frequently. Ensure the vegetables and shrimp are well coated.

Step 6

Season with salt and pepper to taste, top with scallions, and serve immediately.

Step 7

In an airtight container, store leftovers in the refrigerator for up to 3 days.

---

4. Spicy Vegetable Smoothie

Total time: 5 minutes
Servings: 2

Ingredients

- 1 cup coconut water
- 1/2 teaspoon Cayenne powder
- 1 cup baby spinach

- 1 tomato, roughly chopped
- 1 carrot, roughly chopped, frozen
- 1 cucumber, roughly chopped, frozen
- 1 teaspoon garlic, minced
- 1 avocado, fresh or frozen
- 1 lime, peeled

Instructions

Step 1

In a high-speed blender, combine all of the ingredients, then add a pinch of salt. Include both the lime juice and flesh. Blend until smooth.

Step 2

Pour into two serving glasses and serve immediately.

5. Broccoli Salad with Lemon Tahini Sauce

Total time: 35 minutes
Servings: 4

Ingredients

- 6 cups broccoli (about 3-4 large broccoli crowns)
- 1 red onion
- 1 medium-sized cucumber, chopped
- 1/2 cup chopped parsley
- 2 tablespoons hemp seeds
- Juice from 1 large lemon
- 5 tablespoons tahini paste
- 3 tablespoons water
- 3 tablespoons olive oil
- 1 clove minced garlic
- Salt and pepper

Instructions

Step 1

Prepare broccoli by finely chopping and blanching. Chop the red onion, cucumber, and parsley.

Step 2

In a large bowl, combine broccoli, red onion, cucumber, parsley, and hemp seeds.

Step 3

In a separate bowl, combine lemon juice and tahini paste, and whisk using a fork. As you mix, slowly pour in the water. The tahini mixture should coat the back of a spoon once combined.

Step 4

Mix in olive oil and garlic, then season with salt and pepper to your desired taste. Drizzle dressing over the broccoli mixture and mix thoroughly. Best served after 30 minutes to an hour in the fridge to allow flavors to blend.

---

6. Creamy Carrot Ginger Soup

Total time: 25 minutes
Servings: 4

Ingredients

- 4-inch piece fresh ginger peeled and roughly chopped
- 2 cups water
- 2 pounds carrots, washed and chopped
- 1 cup full-fat coconut milk
- 1 medium white onion, chopped
- 3 garlic cloves
- 1 tablespoon ghee
- 1 teaspoon sea salt
- 1/4 cup coconut aminos
- Coconut yogurt
- 2 tablespoons fresh cilantro, chopped
- Raw pumpkin seeds

Instructions

Step 1

In a high-speed blender, combine the ginger and water and blend to produce a "ginger broth." Transfer the broth to a medium, heavy-bottomed pot.

Step 2

Add the carrots, milk, onion, garlic, ghee, salt, and coconut aminos and stir to incorporate. Turn the heat to high and bring it to a boil. Reduce to low heat, cover, and simmer for 12 minutes, or until the carrots are softened.

Step 3

Turn off the heat, uncover, and set aside for 10 to 15 minutes to cool.

Step 4

Pour the soup into a blender. Begin blending on low and gradually increase to high speed until the soup is silky smooth. Alternatively, use a handheld immersion blender to purée the soup right in the pot.

Step 5

If needed, reheat the soup. Pour half of the soup into a small pot and heat on low for a few minutes.

Step 6

Serve the soup in bowls with a dollop of coconut yogurt, cilantro, and pumpkin seeds on top.

7. Easy Bruschetta Salad

Total time: 5 minutes
Servings: 2

Ingredients

- 1/4 red onion
- 2 spring onions, white and light green parts only
- 2 cups cherry tomatoes
- 1 handful parsley
- 1 drizzle olive oil
- Salt and pepper to taste

Instructions

Step 1
Chop red onion, spring onion, cherry tomatoes, and parsley and mix in a bowl.

Step 2

Drizzle with olive oil and season to taste with salt and pepper.

That's all! Enjoy!

---

8. Slow-Cooker Brownies

> Total time: 3 hours
> Servings: 16

Ingredients

- 3 eggs
- 1/4 cup coconut oil
- 1/3 cup rice malt syrup
- 1/4 cup coconut flour
- 2 tablespoons cacao powder
- 1/2 teaspoon vanilla extract
- 1/4 teaspoon baking powder
- 1/4 teaspoon Ground Ceylon cinnamon
- 1.8 oz dark chocolate, chopped (85% cacao)

- 7.1 oz sweet potato/yam, cooked, skin removed, and pureed

Instructions

Step 1

Grease the inside of your slow cooker and line it with baking paper halfway up the sides.

Step 2

In a bowl, incorporate all the dry ingredients.

Step 3

In another bowl, whisk together the eggs, coconut oil, rice malt syrup, and sweet potato puree.

Step 4

Mix the dry components into the wet components well.

Step 5

Pour into the slow cooker and spread it out evenly.

Step 6

Cook for two hours on low or one hour on high.

Step 7

Remove the lid and cook for another 30 minutes or until a skewer inserted into the middle comes out clean.

---

9. Trail Mix

Total time: 25 minutes
Servings: 12

Ingredients

- 1 cup cashew nuts
- 1 cup pecans
- 1 cup almonds
- 1 1/2 cups coconut flakes
- 1 tablespoon Stevia/Monk Fruit erythritol blend
- 1/2 teaspoon Ground Ceylon cinnamon
- 1/2 teaspoon salt
- 1 tablespoon coconut oil (melted)
- 100g chocolate bar, chopped (85%-90% cacao)

Instructions

Step 1

Preheat the oven to 325°F (165°C) and line a baking sheet with parchment paper.

Step 2

In a mixing bowl, combine all of the ingredients, except the chocolate, and season with a pinch of salt to taste. Toss everything together, then spread it on a baking sheet.

Step 3

Bake for 15 minutes, stirring once halfway through.

Step 4

Allow to cool after removing from the oven. Add the chopped chocolate and stir to incorporate.

Step 5

In an airtight container, store in a cool, dry place, for up to 4 weeks.

10. Baked Zucchini Chips

Total time: 3 hours
Servings: 2

Ingredients

- ❖ 2 zucchinis
- ❖ 1 tablespoon olive oil
- ❖ 1 teaspoon salt

Instructions

Step 1

Preheat the oven to 200°F (100°C) and line two baking sheets with parchment paper. Ensure to use parchment paper for this recipe because it helps the chips become crispy on the bottom.

Step 2

Thinly slice the zucchini with a mandolin slicer to 1/16 - 1/8" (1.5 - 3 mm) thickness.

Step 3

Place the zucchini in a bowl, drizzle with olive oil, and toss gently to coat.

Step 4

Arrange the zucchini slices on the baking sheets closely together (but not touching). Season with salt to taste and any additional spices you want to try. While plain salted zucchini chips are delicious, additional flavor combinations to try include smoked paprika and garlic; or basil, oregano, and red pepper flakes. Remember that the spices will become more concentrated as the zucchini shrinks in the oven, so just a small sprinkling is required.

Step 5

Place in the oven and bake for 2 to 2 1/2 hours or until crisp and golden. Once done, turn off the heat and prop open the oven door. Allow the zucchini to cool for another 30 minutes in the warm oven.

Serve on its own or with your favorite dip.